MW00947143

A Guide to Juicing, Raw Foods & Superfoods

Eat a Healthy Diet & Lose Weight

by

Geoff & Vicky Wells

Published by Geezer Guides

Copyright 2013 Geoff & Vicky Wells

ISBN-13: 978-1482791273

ISBN-10: 1482791277

TABLE OF CONTENTS

PUBLISHERS NOTES

DISCLAIMER

This publication is intended to provide helpful and informative material. It is not intended to diagnose, treat, cure, or prevent any health problem or condition, nor is intended to replace the advice of a physician. No action should be taken solely on the contents of this book. Always consult your physician or qualified health-care professional on any matters regarding your health and before adopting any suggestions in this book or drawing inferences from it.

The author and publisher specifically disclaim all responsibility for any liability, loss or risk, personal or otherwise, which is incurred as a consequence, directly or indirectly, from the use or application of any contents of this book.

Any and all product names referenced within this book are the trademarks of their respective owners. None of these owners have sponsored, authorized, endorsed, or approved this book.

Always read all information provided by the manufacturers' product labels before using their products. The author and publisher are not responsible for claims made by manufacturers.

PAPERBACK EDITION 2013

Manufactured in the United States of America

DEDICATION

This book is dedicated to the documentary film makers working to enlighten us all to the abuses of the corporate food industry, government regulatory agencies and agribusiness chemical companies.

If you want to find out more about the move to a natural wholesome diet there are a few documentaries that we think you will enjoy. You will find most of them on the US version of Netflix. Because of licensing restrictions some may not be available where you live, (unless you log into Netflix through a VPN connection).

We have included the website for each of the documentaries where you can either watch them or purchase a DVD.

- ❖ Hungry For Change - http://www.hungryforchange.tv/
- ❖ Forks Over Knives - http://www.forksoverknives.com/
- ❖ Food Inc - http://www.takepart.com/foodinc
- ❖ The Gerson Miracle - http://gerson.org/gerpress/
- ❖ Food Matters - http://www.foodmatters.tv/
- ❖ Fresh - http://www.freshthemovie.com/
- ❖ Food Fight - http://www.foodfightthedoc.com/
- ❖ Ingredients - http://www.ingredientsfilm.com/
- ❖ Fat, Sick & Nearly Dead - http://www.fatsickandnearlydead.com/
- ❖ Dirt! The Movie - http://www.thedirtmovie.org/
- ❖ Vegucated - http://www.getvegucated.com/
- ❖ Tapped - http://www.tappedthemovie.com/
- ❖ Simply Raw Reversing Diabetes - http://www.rawfor30days.com/themovie.html
- ❖ One Man, One Cow, One Planet - http://onemanonecow.com/
- ❖ Genetic Roulette - http://geneticroulettemovie.com/

INTRODUCTION

Thank you for purchasing our book. We hope you will find it interesting and if you decide to follow our recommendations we are sure you will benefit from a healthier, longer life.

We are both in our sixties and have struggled with our weight all our lives. Geoff weighed 158lbs when he was only eleven years old and was considered the school fat kid. This was back before the current obesity epidemic when fat kids were not the norm.

We had pretty much resigned ourselves to the fact that we would remain overweight for the rest of our lives. One day we watched a documentary on Netflix called "Food Inc." It was a life changing moment. We started doing more research into how we were being poisoned by the chemical and food conglomerates. The result was a drastic change in our diet, dramatic weight loss, more energy and vitality. Best all WE WERE NOT HUNGRY!

The information in this book is important for everyone because we are what we eat. Even if you don't fully adopt the practices we recommend we hope you will at least strive to incorporate more healthy food into your diet,

If you do decide this is the lifestyle you have been searching for don't be too obsessive. Indulging in a craving once in a while is OK and won't wreck your diet, just don't let the odd craving turn into a habit.

A Candid Interview With The Authors:

You've said that you're "reluctant" vegetarians. What factors made you choose a mostly vegetarian diet?

Geoff

I had always seen vegetarians and vegans as kind of "out there" and even wackos. I, too, had been taken in by the idea that the only way you could get enough protein was to eat meat.

I found a lot of documentaries for us to watch about the safety of our food. It also highlighted the horrible cruelty to food animals. Even though some of these are really difficult to watch, everyone should know where their food comes from. After watching these documentaries we felt we really needed to look at a better, safer way of eating.

Vicky

Yes, some of the documentaries were difficult to watch, but this is stuff we all need to know. I shed several tears watching how horribly food animals were treated. And - I didn't know that food animals are not covered by any of the animal cruelty laws. Seeing how food animals are treated is shocking and abuse is not a strong enough word. I don't want to contribute to that kind of cruelty.

What did you find the most challenging when you decided to become vegetarians?

Vicky

At first I found meal planning pretty challenging. My normal mode of meal planning consisted of "What meat are we going to have?" followed by "Ok, what goes well with that kind of meat?". When we removed meat from the equation I felt kind of lost and overwhelmed, at first.

What prompted you to write this book?

Geoff

We noticed how there was a lot of confusion and misinformation out there. And, we had been sucked in by a lot of it. As we switched to a healthier, plant-based diet, we found ourselves sorting through all kinds of information, misinformation and some downright lies.

We want to share what we've learned and to share that there is no one "superfood", no magic diet. You don't have to eat all raw, or juice everything. We have found that it's a combination of everything - plant-based foods, raw foods, juicing and, yes, even super foods. It doesn't have to be complicated. You just need a good variety of good food.

Have you seen any specific benefits, personally, since switching to a mostly plant-based diet?

VICKY

I've always had problems controlling my weight, ever since I was a teenager. I had resigned myself to the fact that, if I wanted to be slim, I would simply have to starve myself - and sometimes that didn't even seem to work. Now the weight is coming off all by itself. I'm amazed. I'm not counting calories. I'm not weighing or measuring anything. I'm just sticking to a mostly plant-based diet and making sure I don't add too much fat. Mostly I use olive oil or coconut oil, but sparingly. Anyway, the weight has just been coming off on its own - so far over 20 pounds!

Also, and I didn't even realize this until Geoff mentioned it, but I used to have a terrible time with acid reflux. Almost always, right after eating, I'd get that awful heartburn and reflux. I didn't dare lay down until at least an hour - or more - after eating anything, or even having something to drink. If I did I'd end up choking, sometimes badly, on the reflux coming back up my throat. It was horrible. But after a few weeks of our new way of eating, Geoff asked me about the reflux and I realized that I hadn't had a single episode. Now that's amazing!

GEOFF

Not only that, but we don't feel hungry between meals anymore. We've read that if your body is getting the proper nutrition that you won't feel hungry and, apparently, that's true. We're experiencing exactly that.

Do you choose organic produce?

VICKY

Sometimes getting organic produce can be difficult. In the winters we live on a small Bahamian out-island and in the summers we live in a small Northern

Ontario town. We've found that the best way to get most of our organic produce is to grow it ourselves.

GEOFF

Yes, and growing your own produce can be easier than you think. If your space is limited, think container gardening. We have a little more space, so we like to use raised-bed gardening. We often produce enough to freeze sufficient amounts to see us through the non-growing seasons. And the taste of food you have grown yourself is incredible. If you only buy produce from grocery stores, which may be a week or more old, taste something that's only just been picked and you won't believe the difference. When we harvested our first homegrown carrots, we just scrubbed off the dirt and bit into them. We couldn't believe the wonderful, sweet taste. Nothing like the ones you get in those cello packs.

Was it difficult to eliminate meat from your diet?

VICKY

I certainly thought it was going to be. It's been a big part of my meals for years. Once I got past the meal planning dilemma I found that I didn't really miss the meat at all. Now, when I see recipe pictures that prominently feature meat, with only a few veggies, almost as an afterthought, I find them lacking and uninspiring.

GEOFF

We're not obsessive about being vegetarian. If we really wanted some meat we would have it but after a while you just don't want it.

Are you afraid of being labeled as eccentric or even wackos?

GEOFF

We'll never be what we consider "woo-woo" types. Don't look for us to include crystals and such in our quest for better health. We simply wanted to eat a healthier diet in order to improve our own health and fitness. And … we want to be able to share what we learn so others are able to sort out the fact from fiction.

VICKY

That's right. We're just not "over the top" types at all. However, this new, healthier way of eating is certainly working for us.

Do you have any guilty pleasures when you don't follow your own advice?

GEOFF

I have always loved cheese. Even as a kid I would rather have a piece of cheese than candy. That's not likely to change. Now instead of having an almost daily cheese sandwich I have a small piece of cheese once in a while with some grapes, apple or pear slices.

VICKY

My guilty pleasure is white bread. Yes, I know, bad - bad - bad. I make all our own bread and do some stunning whole grain breads. I'm also experimenting with gluten free bread recipes. However, from time to time, I just have to have a piece of homemade white bread. And my favorite is the end crust, toasted. As long as I don't do it too often, I figure I'll give myself a pass.

WHAT IS JUICING?

In a world filled with new ideas and lots of new technologies don't be surprised that there are a number of ways to take an old idea and turn it into something exciting and healthy.

Today's easy-to-swallow, healthy topic is all about juicing. What exactly is juicing? Ask five people this question and you will most likely get five different answers that may sound different but essentially say the same thing. Juicing, in simple terms, is finding a way to get the most out of a variety of fruits and vegetables by liquefying all or part of the specific food source.

Juicing was an entirely different process during our great-grandparents days, many moons ago. In those days it was entirely a hands-on process using some type of handheld juicing device. There were no plugs or electricity involved - just a basic and simple metal or wooden tool with a standard template designed to fit the interior of almost any orange, lemon or lime. This antique or vintage kitchen tool came in handy for getting the delicious, juicy goodness out of all kinds of citrus fruits. Sure, a few seeds and a little pulp of the tangy fruits might sneak into that ice cold glass of fruit juice, but it was a small price to pay.

If there was a down side to be found with these good, old-fashioned hand juicers it might be their minimal and simplistic design which left plenty of room for improvement. Hands would get tired from the constant pressure, pushing and squeezing to render the most amount of juice possible. It could take several complete fruits per person to get one whole glass of juice. A lengthy process for sure; but that is the way it was done and people loved the end results. Drinking fresh orange juice or fresh lemonade meant a cool treat with plenty of vitamins the body needed.

Fresh foods were always top on the list and were never considered uncommon. Freshly squeezed juices were often considered a neighborly gesture for friends and visitors. Juicing was here to stay; but would progressively evolve. While these juicing tools were great for their time, they eventually found a way into historical memories instead of futuristic kitchen drawers.

Handheld juicers soon graduated to a more convenient design using hydraulics. The same basic juicing cavity was later designed to be gentler on hands. An incorporated hydraulic handle did the work of applying more pressure to the fruit while a container placed below the fruit held the squeezed juice. Ultimately this saved time and energy, and remained a kitchen staple for years. Some kitchens today still have these styles of juicers.

Moving the hands of time forward allowed the world to see many juicers come and go. Today's hip and technologically savvy juicers are often stylish, juice-producing dynamos practically designed with juicing brains of their own. These juicing machines are prepared to impress owners with exceptional appearance, the fanciest features and large quantities of delicious juices with outstanding health benefits to boot. Now that we have apparently reached the juicing machine Mecca of the 21st century, what else is there to appreciate about juicing? Let's take a good look.

Today, juicing is an incredibly easy, delicious and nutritiously smart way to incorporate both health benefits and flavor into our bodies quickly and safely. Long gone are the days of juicing only oranges and lemons, too. If you haven't discovered the popular juicing bandwagon, it's time to see what all the commotion is about and jump aboard.

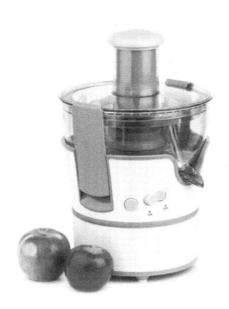

Health and fitness have become the number one people-popularity-winner of the last century. Millions, if not billions of people are vying for the fountain of youth. It comes as no surprise that juicing has soared to the heights of the health improvement revolution. So, how does one actually go about juicing?

Juicing Guide: Enjoying A Raw Food Diet with Superfoods

Beginning with baby steps is always a great way to start something new. Grab your favorite blender. Choose some delicious fruits and/or veggies. Combine all your favorites, cut into smaller pieces for easier blending, place them in your blender and select the liquefy/puree setting. Be sure to remove seeds and stems prior to blending. Pour and enjoy. The downside to some blenders is poor quality blending. Your "liquefied" end result could be a little chunky, although every bit as nutritious and tasty.

If you prefer a more advanced machine, there are several available that actually liquefy the whole food, seeds, skins and all. This is the best choice for juicing and retaining all of the nutritional values nature packed it with in the first place. If you prefer not to juice skins and seeds, simply peel and slice to your liking prior to blending. This method will result in less fiber and nutritional value, however.

Juicing is meant to be fun and delicious. Almost any fruit or veggie can be juiced. Mix and match fruits with veggies for original blends your taste buds will love. Radishes, carrots, apples, cilantro, celery, beets, ginger, you name it, it can all be thrown into the mix of liquefied health in a pitcher.

Don't stop with just fruits and veggies when juicing. Add your favorite herbs and spices, sweeteners, ice cubes and anything else you might like. The whole point of juicing is to create both delicious and healthy recipes. Make ahead enough of your favorite juices to last for several days for convenient, on-the-go nutrition. To keep juices at their peak place them in a dark container, away from light to preserve their nutritional values. Keep chilled in the fridge for quick and easy snacking. A healthy body is as close as your refrigerator door.

Try to remember that juicing is a simple process. Keeping your juices free of any artificial ingredients is healthier and is one of the main goals when juicing. In today's fast and furious world where almost anything goes, go ahead and dive in. Make it your own! You only live once!

Geoff & Vicky Wells

WHAT IS A RAW FOOD DIET?

The raw food diet is a low calorie diet that is similar to a vegan or vegetarian diet. This has been trending lately for people who want to lose weight, improve their health, or want to help the environment in another way. Now why is choosing the raw food diet so much more beneficial than other diets? It is simple; most diets involve you cutting back on food causing you to feel hungry. A raw food diet is packed with healthy nutrition which helps you to feel full. Raw food provides nutrients that help the body reach ultimate nutrition. As food plays a major role in weight loss, the healthier the better!

This might be trending now, but how long has it really been around? The whole raw food movement has been traced all the way back to the late 1800's. Since then science has proven that it really works. It all started with Dr. Maximilian Bircher-Benner. It is claimed that he cured his own disease by eating raw apples. This led to more exciting and new experiments on the phenomena. Nowadays the raw food diet has expanded, quickly. Raw food is exactly what it sounds like. That means it has not been cooked or processed in any shape or form.

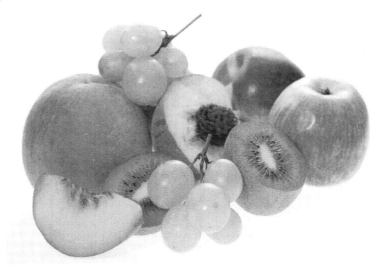

Because it is raw you might be curious as to what types of foods are available for consumption? Simply, fresh fruits, veggies, berries, nuts, seeds, and even some herbs. This gives you a whole range of food to choose from. Why raw though? It has been proven that cooking takes away a lot of the natural vitamins the food produces. Most people on this diet only end up consuming maybe half of what they used to. This sounds drastic but with such healthy food and nutrients going through your body, hunger is not an issue.

Most of the people who choose this diet are vegan, which does not mean you have to eliminate the consumption of other food items. This diet has been modified to suit the individuals' needs. There is no right or wrong, unless your food is heated over 115 degrees, then it is not considered raw anymore. If you do not choose to be vegan and do this you can still consume dairy products.

Here is a small list of the type of foods included in the raw food diet:

❖ Fresh Fruit

❖ Vegetables

❖ Sprouts

❖ Seeds

❖ Nuts

❖ Grains

Many people have even opted to use juicing as a form of raw dieting. This is a good way to include multiple veggies or fruits in one swoop. There is always the question of whether or not you will lose weight. You are likely going to be cutting your food intake in half so there must be some results, right? Yes, you are more likely to lose weight, as long as you are following the raw diet rules. It has been proven that people on this diet weigh a lot less as opposed to someone who isn't. Another benefit of the raw food diet is that it is a great way to keep your blood pressure down. This all seems so good, is there a catch? Nope - no catch. It is ultimately up to you to follow a sensible diet plan that keeps you healthy. A raw food diet gives you access to an amazing number of foods to choose from, so keeping it interesting shouldn't be too difficult.

There are so many health benefits to a raw food diet. You will still get all the protein, carbs, calcium, and fiber your body needs. With healthy eating comes a healthy body. That is why this diet is so popular. Although it can sometimes be hard to follow this diet because it seems like such a drastic change, giving some extra thought to interesting meal preparation can make the transition much more enjoyable and a lot easier, too.

Some people might not enjoy the fact that this is not a convenient diet. Chances are you will not find raw food choices on the menus at most restaurants. Also, you want to make sure that you purchase organic produce whenever possible. With fresh, raw, organic food, taste should never be an issue, as this kind of food is bursting with flavor. And, as you are the one preparing the meals, you can make sure it is to your liking.

For many this an easy transition, but for others, they may be a bit leery about the cost of an organic, whole food diet. Admittedly it can get a little pricey. However, as the saying goes, you get what you pay for. Good quality often commands a higher price. Although choosing organic produce is best, you must also keep your budget in mind. It's better to choose some non-organic items than to abandon a raw food diet altogether based solely on cost. And, don't forget, you won't be purchasing meat at all, which will help to keep your costs in check. This diet was built around the idea of healthy living through plant-based nutrition. And, even though you will lose weight on this diet, that does not mean you should ignore regular exercise. If you've learned anything from trying multiple diets it's that the food helps but if you want to get somewhere you have to move. Exercise and raw healthy eating are ideal for a healthy lifestyle.

Choosing to adopt a raw diet is not as difficult or as scary as it may seem. Just like any diet, you have to make some changes to see progress. While there are never any guarantees, by eating a raw diet you'll cut your caloric intake and, therefore, weight loss should follow. You will also be lessening your risk of heart disease and chronic illnesses. This diet is not for everyone. However, once you have mastered every aspect of the diet including what foods to eat, budgeting and food preparation, this diet should be easy to stick to. It just takes time, a bit of willpower and the knowledge that you're doing the right thing for your health.

Do I Eat Nothing But Raw Food?

It wouldn't hurt you and you would certainly be healthier for it but, no the idea is to incorporate lots of raw food into your diet - at least 50%. Cooked food will have less nutrients than raw food but you also have to consider the quality of your life. Many foods can't be eaten raw. Potatoes, yams, parsnips, beets come to mind but the list may not be that long after all.

WHAT ARE SUPERFOODS?

The term Superfoods is a classification of specific foods and food groups that are beneficial to your health. Today's diets often consist of many unhealthy foods, commonly called "junk" foods, which can have adverse effects on the body's performance, contribute to illness and disease and rob the body of nutrients. Unsafe hybridized and GMO (Genetically Modified Organism) foods and agricultural production are just a few of the culprits when examining today's substandard dietary practices. Heart disease has been attributed to poor nutrition, along with cancer and diabetes, with diabetes the most wide-spreading disease on the globe.

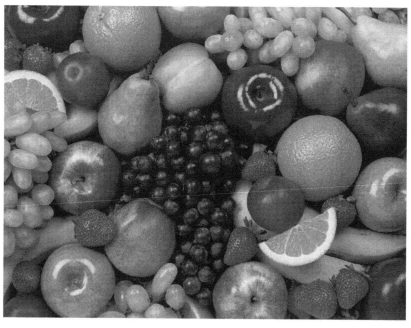

Superfood diets add essential minerals and vitamins to promote maximum nutrition, which is essential in bone, tissue, nerve and muscle development. Superfoods exist in all food groups and excel in delivering the highest health benefits to combat illness and disease. They promote better health by reducing or eliminating any deficiency that might be caused by most normal diet regimes. They are known to fortify the immune system and promote healthy weight loss since they are whole foods and generally either fat-free or low-fat. Changing to a superfood diet has many positive effects, most importantly the health benefits, but it can be fun and interesting when choosing foods that are new to your diet and lifestyle.

The Science Behind It

The wonder of Superfoods is all about the chemicals in the nutrients and their reaction inside the human body. The foods are as variable as the effects they produce. Fish and meat contain high concentrations of proteins and beneficial nutrients. Other sources include turkey, watercress, spinach, yoghurt and broccoli. Nuts and grains, like walnuts and oats make the list. Vegetables and fruits are high on the list since they contain liberal amounts of vitamin C and antioxidants.

Darker fruits contain flavonoids, beta carotene and phytochemicals, which accelerate antioxidant properties. Antioxidants combat harmful molecules known as free radicals, which have proven to be destructive to DNA and human cells and, in their worst form, promote premature aging, cancer and heart disease. Even the lighter colored fruits contain sufficient phytochemicals to make them effective in disease prevention. The nutrients of true Superfoods heighten alertness, energy, vitality, healing and boost the feeling of wellbeing.

Some Highly-Rated Superfoods:

Incan Golden Berries

One of the best snack foods is Incan golden berries, small marble-sized fruits. They can be consumed in raw form, dried or baked in jellies, jams and other dessert forms. They curb hunger and contain almost no calories. They are known for their energizing effects and have a naturally sweet and tangy flavor. The whole berries have a chewy, soft consistency that make them an excellent treat or snack food.

Blue-Green Algae

Blue-green algae has a plethora of phytonutrients, consisting of amino acids, B12, phenyl ethylamine, complex sugars, active enzymes, and glycol proteins. These vitamins and minerals are naturally absorbed very quickly into the body due to their thin and soft cellular walls. The digestive system absorbs and metabolizes all of the beneficial amino and semi-amino acids at close to a 100 percent rate. Blue-green algae scores high as a primary weight loss food, often giving the impression of a full stomach after eating.

Raw Maca

Raw Maca belongs to the family of radishes and cauliflower. Besides beneficial fatty acids, it contains over 20 amino acids and minerals that promote endocrine system maintenance and rejuvenation. Most surprisingly, raw maca is a derivative of the raw cacao bean, otherwise known as chocolate. In its natural and raw form it has high antioxidant vitamin content. Its mineral content is also high, carrying copper, zinc, chromium and magnesium. The unprocessed form is often used as a weight-loss supplement. Eating raw maca can produce a feeling of wellbeing. It also combines well with raw cacao, mushrooms, goji berries, papaya, mango and leafy greens to produce a tasty, low-calorie smoothie drink.

APPLES

Well over 7,500 types of apples are grown worldwide, making accessibility to them easy and affordable. Apples have a natural soluble fiber known as pectin that aids in maintaining a healthy digestive system and helps to reduce high levels of blood cholesterol. They have large amounts of antioxidants and vitamin C, essential for healthy gums and skin. Apples are low on the glycemic index and contain healthy, complex carbohydrates. Since apples break down slowly in the digestive system, they don't spike glucose in the bloodstream. Apples are even sometimes prescribed for the control of diabetes. They rank very high as a fast and convenient snack food. Pears also fall into this fruit category, delivering similar nutritional results.

BROCCOLI

Broccoli, along with cabbage, kale, cauliflower, collards, Brussels sprouts and mustard greets all contain varying amounts of vitamin C, antioxidants and folate. Folate is the natural form of folic acid. The folic acid in broccoli has been shown to reduce the risk of heart disease. Broccoli shows positive benefits in combating cancer, due to its content of sulphoraphane, one of the phytochemicals. Lutein, found in broccoli, helps to prevent AMD, or age related macular degeneration. The effect of AMD is found in approximately 10 percent in the population of persons over the age of 60.

VIRGIN OLIVE OIL

Virgin olive oil, although slightly high in calories, contains a mono saturated fat that benefits the heart. It also reduces bad cholesterol and increases the levels of good cholesterol. In addition to that, it also carries high levels of polyphenols, phytoserols and Vitamin E. Although it is best used at room temperature, a little goes a long way when sautéing or frying foods, since it does not burn off as readily as butter.

BLUEBERRIES

Blueberries, belonging to the family of purple grapes, raspberries, strawberries, blackberries, cherries, cranberries and other frozen or fresh berries, are beneficial for healthy skin due to their anthocyanins content. They provide an excellent source of fiber, aiding the digestive system. They have antioxidant cancer-fighting properties and quell hunger pains. Their mineral content is high, containing manganese, potassium, iron, and they provide sources of phytonutrients, polyphenols and folate. Blueberries contain more antioxidants than any other single food. They make an excellent snack alternative.

GREEN TEA

Green tea increases the metabolism thanks to its abundance of flavonoids. This makes it a good choice as a weight-loss supplement and early morning stimulant. The catechin polyphenols and antioxidant content is known for reducing heart disease. Black tea also falls within this category, yielding similar health benefits. Either beverage is a great choice for meals or as a general thirst-quencher.

WHAT ARE THE BENEFITS OF JUICING?

Today, as more and more people are becoming concerned about their health and are trying to move away from processed foods to better dietary choices, juicing has become popular. Far more than a momentary fad, juicing has been around for centuries. It gained some popularity with Jack LaLane's promotion of juicing in the 1950s and 60s, but has taken until today for the mainstream population to understand and embrace its health benefits. So, why should you juice? What are the benefits to you?

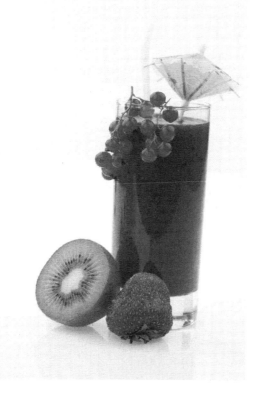

JUICING HELPS BOOST YOUR IMMUNE SYSTEM

No one likes to be sick, and it is no secret that the way to boost your immune system is by consuming the proper amounts of vitamins and minerals. Fruits and vegetable are a rich source of the vitamins and minerals your immune system needs, but it is difficult to eat the required recommended daily amount. While it may be difficult to sit down and eat the recommended 5 to 9 servings of fruits and vegetables a day, when 2 or 3 servings are juiced they can easily fit into a single glass. Also, there are an unlimited number of fruit and/or juice combinations you can use to help keep things interesting.

Juicing Helps Clean Out Your Digestive System

Our digestive system works hard to break down the food we consume each day into microscopic particles and absorb its nutrients. It takes so much work for the digestive system that some food remains in our system undigested. The average person has more than 5 pounds of undigested food in their body at any given time; some people have up to 30. This undigested food, even if it was healthy for you to begin with, becomes toxic to your body, which can lead to serious health issues. When you juice fruits and vegetables, you have already done a good portion of the work for your body. Your body can easily absorb the nutrients from juices leaving your digestive system to work on the food that is still not broken down. This allows you to eliminate the built up toxins, creating a healthier more efficient digestive system.

Juicing Helps You Lose Weight

Another benefit of giving your body the proper amount of nutrients and ridding yourself of toxins is that along with creating a healthier body you are also creating a slimmer one. Simply eliminating all the undigested food from your body results in some weight loss. In addition, since your body is receiving the proper nutrients and calories, it does not store fat like it does in starvation diets. To help enhance weight loss effects, you can always add spices that promote fat burning such as pepper, cinnamon or parsley, which is also an appetite suppressant.

If you are someone who normally craves sweets and other carbohydrates, there are various recipes with tasty combinations of fruits and vegetables that can satisfy your cravings and curb your appetite. Just remember to limit fruits that are high in natural sugars and combine them with vegetables, particularly leafy green vegetables, whenever possible. By doing this you'll get lots of great taste, vitamins and minerals, but less sugar.

Juicing Gives You More Energy

The body is essentially a machine and like any other machine, when properly cared for, it performs better. Most of the food we eat today is like putting low quality gasoline into a performance vehicle; while it may still run, you will not achieve top performance. Fruit and vegetable juices are to the body what performance gasoline is to a car. It makes everything flow better, increasing circulation, which also increases oxygenation, and gives your body what it needs to create more energy.

JUICING HELPS YOU IMPROVE YOUR SKIN AND KEEPS YOU LOOKING YOUNG

Drinking your fruits and vegetable not only gives your skin the nutrients it craves it helps to keep you well hydrated. A study from the University of Witten-Herdecke's Institute for Experimental Dermatology in Germany showed that subjects consuming concentrated fruit juices have increased microcirculation of the skin, more hydration, and an increase in skin thickness and density. While juicing may not turn back the clock 20 years it can help reduce some of the effects that aging has on the skin. There is also evidence to suggest it can help those who suffer from chronic skin conditions like psoriasis. In fact, there are many juice recipes available that were developed to target specific skin conditions.

JUICING GETS EVEN THE PICKIEST CHILD TO CONSUME VEGETABLES

Just ask any mother in the history of the world how hard it can be to get a child to eat their vegetables. The answers will range from difficult to next to impossible. Juicing helps get your children to consume their vegetables because you are masking them. Even just in presentation, a glass of juice to a child is much easier and quicker to consume than a bowl full of carrots. Many children have problems with certain textures, like spinach or kale, but when juiced the texture is no longer a factor.

Not only does it help visually and with the texture, but you can cover up any vegetable tastes they dislike with the sweet taste of fruit flavors. There are many juice recipes available that can make even the most undesirable vegetable palatable to children. With all the ways juice tastes can be manipulated chances are, unless you tell them, most children will never even know they are consuming healthy vegetables. Also, not to be discounted is the fact that most children find a certain cool factor in turning something that is solid into something liquid.

Juicing is really all about integrating healthy, fresh foods into your diet. With modern machines and recipe books, making juicing a part of a healthy lifestyle has never been easier. If you want a healthier lifestyle juicing can be the first step. For those who have already embraced a healthier lifestyle, juicing can be the finishing touch on the important changes you have already made.

WHAT ARE THE BENEFITS OF EATING RAW FOODS?

Eating raw foods has become quite popular and for good reasons. Even if you consume a lot of fruits and vegetables in your diet, if you are cooking them you aren't getting all the nutrients each food has to offer. When you cook your food, you destroy enzymes, many vitamins and proteins. This means that your body is getting fewer nutrients, has to work harder to digest the food and to break down the proteins. With raw foods, you get more nutrients and your body will feel it. There are many benefits to eating raw foods.

WEIGHT LOSS

By eating raw foods, you get all the natural nutrients your body needs. People tend to worry that eating raw foods, like avocados and nuts, that they will gain weight because both foods have high levels of fat. However, by eating all raw foods, you don't have to worry about those fat levels and will easily loose and keep off weight. As long as you don't eat massive amounts of high-fat raw foods, you don't have anything to worry about. Moderation and variety is the key.

BETTER SKIN

Raw foods help to hydrate and oxygenate your cells. This helps to make your skin look great. With a raw food diet, you can stay healthier and looking younger. It is anti-aging without any expensive creams, face lifts or make-up - just natural and healthy eating.

MORE ENERGY

No more afternoon naps! By maintaining a raw diet, you will have more energy to make it through the day. In fact, you will even need less sleep at night. Raw foods allow you to be more alert during the day and sleep better at night, therefore you may find that you need less sleep each night.

LOWER CHOLESTEROL

A diet without all the fat and cholesterol from meat means you will have a healthier body and lower cholesterol. That relates to a lower risk of developing heart or cardiovascular disease. So not only will you lose weight, feel better and look better but you will also be prolonging your life.

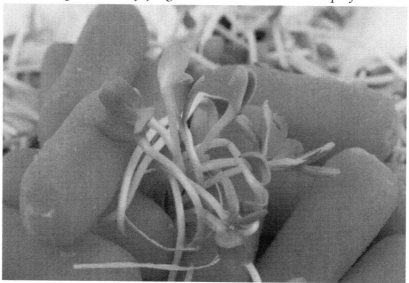

DIGESTION

Although it's not a common topic for discussion, everyone knows that it's good to have regular bowel movements. Regularity is directly related to digestion. When you consume raw foods, you consume a lot of enzymes. This makes digestion easier for your body because the enzymes will help break down the food. Not only does this help you have easier, regular bowel movements but it gives you more energy because you body doesn't have to divert that energy to the digestion process.

MORE TIME

There are many, many health benefits to eating raw foods, but it doesn't stop there. It takes almost no time to prepare raw foods. All you need to do it wash and serve - making it perfect for the busy person or family. With the quick preparation and minimal cleanup you'll have more time for work, friends and family.

YOU CAN EAT A LOT

This is one of our favorite benefits because we do love to eat.

Since raw food is so easy for your body to digest, you can eat almost as much of it as you want. No more counting calories and cutting back just eat all the raw foods you want. But at the same time, because of the fiber and the nutrients, it will take less food to fill you up and keep you full.

SAVES MONEY

Your body will be healthier and stronger on a raw food diet. People think that eating healthy costs too much money however, when you eat healthy, you spend less time sick or at the doctors. This means you don't have to spend money on medical bills or miss time at work. Your grocery bill may be a little more each week but you medical expenses will be way down.

Also, you won't be buying any meat, so that can certainly help to reduce, or offset, any increase in your food costs.

All in all, you could end up saving money when you take all factors into consideration.

ENVIRONMENTALLY FRIENDLY

When you eat raw foods, you are helping both yourself and the earth. There is little to no packaging with raw foods. This means you will have less waste to throw out: less cardboard, less plastic, less tin, etc.

If you purchase organic produce, then there are less harmful chemicals used when the produce is being grown. That also good for both you and the earth.

If you eat little or no meat, then fewer food animals will be raised. That means less methane released into the atmosphere, fewer antibiotics, growth hormones and the like being used on animals (and getting into your food) and less cruelty to animals, too. That's good for everyone, including the animals.

If you want to feel and look great, adopting a raw food diet is an easy to way to accomplish it. When you eat raw foods, you get all the natural nutrients your body needs. Nothing is added, nothing is taken out and it is the just the right amount of everything.

PROTEIN

A lot of people worry about their protein intake while on a raw food diet. But there is nothing to worry about. With the right mix of food, you will get all the protein your body needs to be healthy. In fact, proteins from vegetables are easier for your body to break down than proteins from animals. Protein from animals is full of cholesterol, which is difficult for the body to breakdown. Vegetable protein is easier for the body to absorb and use.

There are so many benefits to eating raw foods. It helps your body feel and look younger while still allowing you to enjoy great tasting foods. You don't have to worry about how much food you eat or how many calories you take in. You will start to lose weight quickly and keep it off. Additionally, if you eat a lot of greens and a variety of raw foods you will get all the protein your body needs.

But the health factors aren't the only good thing. You will save money, help the environment and have more free time. No more scrubbing greasy pans or spending hours cooking dinner. Raw foods are quick, easy and delicious. They don't come in packaging that is harmful to the environment and will help reduce the amount of waste your household creates.

The benefits of raw food are endless. It can help in every aspect of your life: health, family and environment. Don't eat empty calories by cooking the nutrients out of your food - live healthy and eat raw foods.

WHAT ARE THE BENEFITS OF SUPERFOODS?

Everyone is looking for that magic formula that will slow or stop the aging process, defy gravity, provide weight loss and keep them disease free. Sounds complicated and impossible when you really stop to think about it but superfoods can help with all of that and more.

A simple solution is often staring you right in the face, either in your own kitchen or at your local grocery store or farmers market. Nutritionally speaking, Superfoods provide you with more of the nutrients and healthy building blocks to keep your body healthy and running at optimum levels more than any of the regular pre-packaged or overly processed foods could ever do.

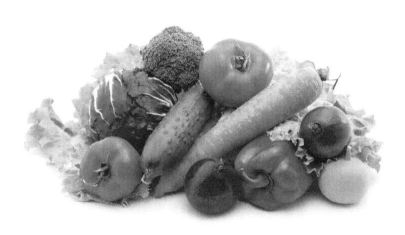

Frequently, superfoods aren't any more expensive than other food items; in fact, many are much more economical than pre-packaged, highly processed, nutritionally void food items. Budget friendly foods that provide all of your nutritional needs are available at local grocery stores, farmers markets and specialty food stores. With such wide availability you would think that everyone would be eating superfoods but, unfortunately, that's not the case.

A healthy diet often results in not only physical wellbeing, but emotional wellbeing as well. If your body is healthy, your mind naturally follows. Striving to keep your entire system in peak performance takes little to no more effort than preparing simple healthy meals like our grandparents used to do. They created most of their meals from scratch using fresh and, most often, locally grown foods.

For anyone dealing with heart disease, asthma, diabetes or seasonal allergies, superfoods can make a huge difference in alleviating, and sometimes eliminating, their problems. Eating healthy needs to be a way of life not just a lifestyle.

Eliminating foods that are overly processed causes your body's natural healing systems to kick in and remove the toxins that have accumulated from such poor quality foods. These changes in turn create a healthier body and can reduce, or eliminate, the symptoms of many medical conditions.

In many cases it's possible to lower high blood pressure by simply eliminating excess salt from your diet. Since most, if not all, packaged foods add sodium, it only stands to reason that switching to fresh, whole superfoods (foods that haven't been pre-packaged and are more nutritionally dense) would help to lower blood pressure.

While Superfoods aren't necessarily a replacement for medications or visits to your doctor, they can certainly improve a lot of medical conditions and, in time, your doctor may reduce or eliminate some medications. Don't rely on any particular food item to replace a medication. Always consult your doctor before stopping or reducing any medication you may be taking.

Although some people many complain that superfoods aren't convenient, many others are finding that, with a few minutes of preparation, it's much easier to have healthy snacks and meals available. Kids love helping themselves to fresh cut fruits and vegetables. Healthy dinners can easily be prepared ahead of time to be cooked in a slow cooker with little mess and fuss.

It's essential to get rid of the junk foods in your home. By doing that no one will be tempted to reach for the junk food and, instead, will have healthy fruits and vegetables to choose from. Kids will not only like this but they will end up with more energy and fewer weight problems. The same goes for you.

There's a lot of buzz about antioxidants right now and that's because they help to increase stamina, decrease the signs of aging and help improve your overall health. Incorporating superfoods into your diet will increase these healthy antioxidants with minimal effort.

For those of us who are looking for the fountain of youth, these foods will not only improve your health but will also help you to feel younger and more energetic. Delicious foods such as oatmeal, pears and avocados, eaten instead of high fat, high sugar cereals and snacks, can have the added benefit of reducing your cholesterol as well.

Diets higher in fiber may improve heart conditions, reduce cholesterol and reduce many types of cancers. Adding fiber to a diet in lieu of overly processed meats is a simple act that may just save a life.

Instead of fat laden French fries you may find that you enjoy oven-baked sweet potato "fries" even more. The sweeter taste also lures in fussy eaters without them even realizing they're exchanging an unhealthy food for a healthier, more nutritious option. Slice up a few sweet potatoes, toss them in a little olive oil and some salt and pepper, and bake them for a healthier alternative to fries. You're likely to fall in love a new taste sensation that's actually good for you.

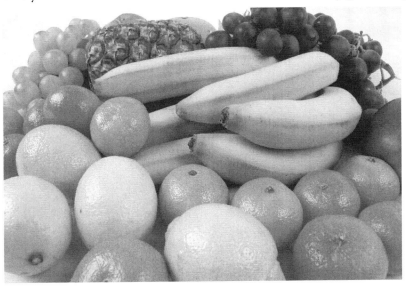

Berries are another superfood that just about everyone loves. Full of antioxidants, phytonutrients and low in calories they may just be the perfect year around food. Great for smoothies (add some Greek yogurt with a handful of frozen berries for a super taste treat), dried and added to oatmeal, dried as a snack, fresh off the vine or just slightly chilled, this wonder food is an amazing addition to any diet.

Superfoods are a great way to detoxify a body. Eliminating toxins that make you feel sluggish and drained and replacing them with healthier alternatives is often the only change you need to feel more energetic. Try a few simple diet changes this week and see how you feel.

A lot of people seem to worry that by switching to a healthy way of eating means giving up all of their favorite foods. This couldn't be further from the truth. Even a chocolate lover can cash in on the benefits of superfoods. Dark chocolate, that isn't overly processed and has high cacao content, can help protect DNA and blood vessels. Adding just one ounce of this incredible food can provide a healthy taste treat for your sweet tooth.

Simple changes, like eliminating all types of soda, whether diet or not, and exchanging it for green tea, will go a long way in protecting your overall health. Try eating a small handful of nuts instead of a candy bar. Use honey or, better yet, real maple syrup, instead of processed sugar, as your sweetener of choice. Both of those sweeteners will introduce a new taste sensation and, did you know that honey is a natural antibiotic?

No, healthy eating is not all rabbit food, rocks and twigs. These foods go back to the basics that our grandparents used to use. In today's society we've become too accustomed to grabbing a quick, processed snack in lieu of healthier alternatives.

Read the labels. If there are a huge number of ingredients and some of them are difficult, or impossible, to pronounce then chances are it's not good for you.

COMBINING IT ALL FOR A HEALTHY LIFESTYLE

When we say "let's combine it all for a healthier lifestyle", this could mean something different to just about everyone. Often we mistakenly believe that if we just go on a diet and get in a couple of hours a week at the gym all will be well. In actuality, combining it all not only refers to a healthy diet and exercise regimen that involves getting active, but also; maintaining good relationships, lowering our stress factors and, of course, getting adequate rest.

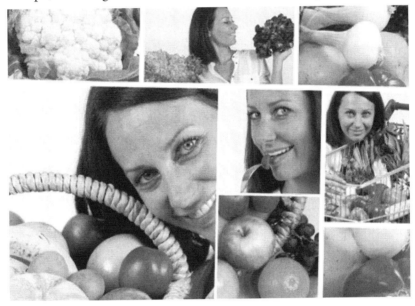

The human body is a complex machine that only runs well on the proper fuels – in other words, proper nutrition from complete foods and not the food-like products that have invaded our lives. A diet rich in fruits, vegetables and proteins is a great way to maintain proper nutrition. Protein, which is readily available from many plant-based foods, is essential for building healthy muscles, teeth and bones.

We are always searching for the right balance. A good place to start your journey towards a balanced, healthy life is to start by adding superfoods to your diet. Superfoods are "nutrient-rich" foods that impart many benefits to your body. Superfoods contain antioxidants, minerals, essential vitamins, amino acids, fatty acids, enzymes and glyconutrients.

These foods are clean, organic and just plain good for you. They help increase your body's immunity, improve eyesight, protect your liver, improve your heart function and blood quality and some of these foods actually help you sleep better, too. A few prime examples of Superfoods are many types of berries such as; acai, blackberries, blueberries and strawberries. Other great tasting Superfoods are spinach, pumpkins, salmon, oats and tomatoes. Superfoods have even been shown to the aid in the fight against certain forms of cancer!

Let's not forget to include all the great natural juices that can be prepared quickly and easily using raw foods like cabbage, kale, lettuce, carrots, melons, berries – the list is almost endless.

As we mentioned, a healthy lifestyle isn't just about eating healthy. Getting active can mean many different things. Working out at the gym whenever you can is always good idea, but often you may just not have the time. There are other, easier ways to fit in some physical activity. Take the stairs instead of the elevator when you can, take part in a competitive sport with a friend or co-worker - things like tennis, racquetball or basketball. Head to the local pool and swim some laps or participate in a water aerobics class. Take your dog out for a walk. If you think about it, there are a million and one ways to stay active. All you have to do is find ways to fit it in to your busy schedule.

When you go to the mall do you struggle to find the parking space closest to the door? You will find lots of empty spaces on the outer rows and get the benefit of a little exercise if you park far away from the door.

Maintaining good relationships and lowering your stress levels often go hand in hand. Having a good relationship with the people around us is just one of the many ways to successfully manage stress. It is no secret that stress is a big cause of many degenerative and chronic health problems. Stress can cause high blood pressure and that can cause artery damage, heart problems or an aneurysm. High blood pressure, left untreated, can also cause kidney scarring and even failure.

The importance of lowering the amount of stress in our lives cannot be overstated. It can, quite literally, be the difference between life and death. We can avoid unnecessary stress simply by making wise choices and learning how not to sweat the small stuff. There is no need to work a long day and bring work stress home. That will only lead to unnecessary arguments and hurt feelings. Avoid excess alcohol and harmful drugs. Make time for yourself and time to spend with your loved ones as well. Take vacations, have date nights, spend time with family and friends. Life is too short to have regrets.

Last, and certainly not least, allow yourself plenty of time for adequate rest.

There are many who claim that they can get by on just a few hours of sleep, but too much or too little is never good. The quality of your sleep is what's important. No one can perform mental tasks well if they are tired! If your sleep gets interrupted or cut short, you're not getting a good quality of sleep. Children and older adults need more sleep than the average adult. Older adults have the tendency to sleep more lightly and wake more frequently. It is important to remember that as you age your sleep patterns will change. Naturally, pregnant women often require more sleep and rest in general. Overall, the average adult who gets roughly seven to nine hours of sleep a night tends to function better. No one is impervious to sleep problems and it is obviously best to consult a doctor if you are not getting the amount of rest you need so they can determine the reasons for your sleeplessness.

So many things play pivotal roles in maintaining a healthy lifestyle. Keeping a positive attitude, getting regular checkups, taking time off, maintaining relationships and, of course, eating healthy, whole foods are all part of the picture. No one thing is going to make, or keep, you healthy. The key is variety, moderation and balance.

VITAMIX

Before we get to the recipes we thought we should say something about the tools you need, in particular the blender or juicer that is best for the job.

We have owned juicers in the past and found them to be a pain to clean, particularly the centrifugal type that spin the pulp against a mesh that has to be cleaned.

This is not a VitaMix commercial but that is what we currently use and we love it. It can handle everything we throw at it and it is a breeze to clean.

The Vitamix is a commercial blender - the type they use at Orange Julius juice stands. It is way more expensive than an ordinary domestic blender but you get what you pay for.

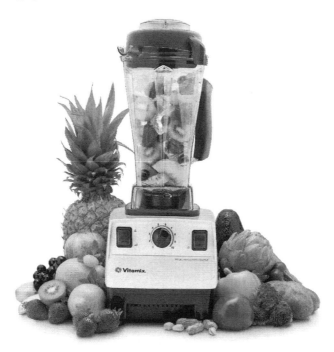

There are several different models and you can get them from Amazon, Costco or a product demonstration at shows and exhibits across the country.

THE RECIPES

We know that when you transition to a mostly plant-based diet that you're going to be looking for a lot of recipes.

Here's a few of our favorites that we have developed over the last little while.

Most of these use raw foods and, of course, superfoods. Lots of them are juicing and/or smoothies recipes.

As we researched recipes for our newfound, healthy lifestyle, we found that we were adding, or subtracting, ingredients to create meals that suited our own preferences. We encourage you to do the same.

We particularly like being able to make our own nut milks and find them so much better than the commercially produced ones.

We have included a few other recipes, too, like Multi-Bean Salad and Granola, to try to round things out a bit.

We're constantly developing new recipes. Some are wonderful and we hope to share those in other books or on our website. Others belong in the "Well, I won't try that again" category. Aren't you glad we eliminated those ones for you?

The whole idea is to experiment and explore new taste experiences while transitioning to a healthier life.

We've created a new website for this book and others we hope to add to the series - we hope you will check it out.

http://reluctantvegetarians.com/

Enjoy!

ALMOND MILK

Who knew that making your own almond milk could be this easy? We've been doing this for a while and almost never buy the commercially produced type now.

INGREDIENTS

> 1 cup raw almonds
> 3 cups filtered water
> sugar, to taste, optional

METHOD

Place the almonds, water and sugar (if using) in the blender.

Make sure that lid is secure and begin blending at lowest speed increasing gradually to maximum speed.

Blend for at least two minutes or until smooth.

If desired, filter the almond milk through a fine mesh sieve to remove any sediment or grit.

Store in the refrigerator.

SERVINGS: 7

Baby Spinach Salad

Spinach is another plant that seems to grow well in our garden. We make a lot of spinach salads when it's in season.

Ingredients

    2 cups baby spinach leaves, packed
    1 large pear
    1 teaspoon lemon juice, freshly squeezed
    ½ cup chickpeas
    ¼ cup cashew halves
    2 tablespoons raisins or craisins
    4 tablespoons extra virgin olive oil
    3 tablespoons apple cider vinegar
    2 tablespoons maple syrup
    1 sprig fresh rosemary
    sea salt, to taste
    black pepper, freshly ground, to taste

Method

Wash the spinach well and spin or pat dry.

Wash the pear, cut it in quarters, core it and coarsely chop it. Toss the chopped pear in the lemon juice to prevent it from going brown.

In a large salad bowl, combine the spinach, pear, chickpeas, cashews and raisins. Toss to mix.

In a separate bowl, whisk together the olive oil, vinegar and maple syrup. Remove the leaves from the sprig of Rosemary and add them to the oil and vinegar mixture. Whisk again. Add the salt and pepper to taste and whisk once more.

Gently pour the oil and vinegar mixture over the salad and toss lightly to combine.

Serve immediately.

Servings: 2

BANANA, MELON, CARROT JUICE

We are having lots of fun - and nutrition - exploring all the amazing foods you can put in a juice or a smoothie. This one is lovely and sweet.

INGREDIENTS

> 1 medium banana, ripe
> ½ cup cantaloupe, chunks
> ¼ cup carrots, coarsely chopped
> ½ medium kiwi, peeled
> ¼ cup orange segments
> ¼ small lemon, peeled
> 1 tablespoon honey
> ⅛ teaspoon nutmeg, optional
> ½ cup pineapple chunks
> ½ cup water
> 1 cup ice cubes

METHOD

Place all ingredients in the blender.

Make sure that lid is secure and begin blending at lowest speed increasing gradually to maximum speed.

Blend for at least one minute or until everything is well blended and smooth.

Serve immediately.

SERVINGS: 2

CASHEW MILK

We find cashews naturally sweet, so we don't add any sugar, but you may want to. Why not try it without first? You can always sweeten it later.

INGREDIENTS

>   1 cup raw cashews
>   3 cups filtered water
>   sugar, to taste, optional

METHOD

Place all ingredients in the blender.

Make sure that lid is secure and begin blending at lowest speed increasing gradually to maximum speed.

Blend for at least two minutes or until smooth.

Cashew milk does not require filtering. Store it in the refrigerator and shake well before using.

SERVINGS: 7

Chocolate and Coconut Smoothie

Chocolate and coconut go so well together. Be sure to see how to make your own coconut milk recipe in this book. That way you can use your own, homemade coconut milk in this recipe.

Ingredients

1 cup coconut milk
1 tablespoon raw cacao
4 Medjool dates
1 medium banana, fresh or frozen
1 cup ice cubes

Method

Place all ingredients in the blender in the order given.

Make sure that lid is secure and begin blending at lowest speed increasing gradually to maximum speed.

Blend for at least one minute or until everything is well blended and smooth.

Serve immediately.

Servings: 2

Geoff & Vicky Wells

EYE OPENER SMOOTHIE

A great morning smoothie - no sweetener required.

We've used a Vitamix commercial grade blender to make this smoothie. If you're using a non-commercial grade blender, be sure to cut things up into smaller chunks so you don't overload the blender.

INGREDIENTS

1½ cups almond milk
1 cup kale, packed
1 small orange, peeled
1 small pear, quartered and seeded
1 small apple, quartered and seeded
1 cup honeydew melon , chunks
1 medium banana, fresh or frozen
1 tablespoon ground flax seed
1 teaspoon diatomaceous earth, food grade, optional

METHOD

Place all ingredients in the blender in the order given.

Make sure that lid is secure and begin blending at lowest speed increasing gradually to maximum speed.

Blend for at least one minute or until everything is well blended and smooth.

Serve immediately.

SERVINGS: 2

Fresh From The Garden Vegetable Cocktail

We both love a nice glass of garden cocktail with our lunch most days. Now that we're growing a lot of our own produce, we can make it fresh from the garden. The taste is amazing!

INGREDIENTS

3 medium tomatoes, quartered
½ cup lettuce leaves, torn
1 stalk celery, including leaves
¼ cup carrots, coarsely chopped
1 spring onions, sliced
¼ cup red bell pepper, coarsely chopped
2 sprigs parsley
⅛ teaspoon tabasco sauce, optional
½ teaspoon soy sauce, optional
1 dash sea salt, optional
1 dash freshly ground black pepper, optional
1 cup ice cubes

METHOD

Place all of the ingredients in the blender.

Make sure that lid is secure and begin blending at lowest speed increasing gradually to maximum speed.

Blend for at least one minute or until all ingredients are smooth and well blended.

Serve immediately.

SERVINGS: 2

FROSTY CARROT JUICE

Truly fresh carrots are just naturally sweet. This frosty carrot drink is refreshing and tasty.

INGREDIENTS

- 1½ cups carrots, coarsely chopped
- 1 cup water
- 2 teaspoons freshly squeezed lemon juice
- 1 cup ice cubes

METHOD

Place all of the ingredients in the blender.

Make sure the lid is secure and start at the lowest speed, gradually increasing to maximum speed.

Blend for one minute or until everything is smooth and well blended.

Service immediately.

SERVINGS: 2

Geoff's Famous Hummus

Geoff loves to experiment with hummus recipes and this is his "famous" recipe. Very, very tasty.

Ingredients

    1 can chickpeas, 15 ounces, drained, reserve liquid
    1 ounce sun dried tomatoes, not packed in water or oil
    ½ lime, juice only
    3 cloves garlic
    6 slices jalapeno, or to taste
    3 teaspoons tahini paste
    ½ teaspoon sea salt
    ½ teaspoon freshly ground black pepper
    1 tablespoon balsamic vinegar

Method

Place all ingredients, in order listed, in a food processor and blend until smooth.

Add reserved liquid as required to achieve desired consistency. You'll probably need about half of the liquid.

Servings: 24

GOODNESS GRACIOUS GREEN

What a great way to get your greens! This one is good for any time of the day, even as a snack.

INGREDIENTS

    1 head broccoli, coarsely chopped
    ¼ cup kale, packed
    ¼ cup baby spinach, packed
    1 stalk celery, including leaves
    ½ cup carrots, coarsely chopped
    ½ green apple, coarsely chopped
    ½ cup water
    1 cup ice cubes

METHOD

Place all ingredients in the blender.

Make sure the lid is secure and start at the lowest speed, gradually increasing to maximum speed.

Blend for at least one minute or until all ingredients are smooth and well blended.

Serve immediately.

SERVINGS: 3

Hot Tomato Drink

Our garden just loves to produce tomatoes - in abundance - so we often make this hot drink. But, even if you don't want it hot right from the blender, you can always freeze the juice for later use.

INGREDIENTS

    1 cup tomato, coarsely chopped
    ½ tablespoon freshly squeezed lemon juice
    ½ vegetable bouillon cube, optional
    ⅛ teaspoon dry mustard, optional
    ⅛ teaspoon sea salt
    ⅛ teaspoon freshly ground black pepper
    2 sprigs parsley
    ½ cup boiling water

METHOD

Combine all ingredients in the blender, adding the boiling water last.

Make sure the lid is secure and start at the lowest speed, gradually increasing to maximum speed.

Blend for two to three minutes or until everything is smooth and well blended.

Servie immediately.

SERVINGS: 1

HOT VEGGIE DRINK

Similar to the garden cocktail, this drink can be served hot from the blender, cooled or even frozen for later use.

INGREDIENTS

2 large tomato, coarsely chopped
1 stalk celery, including leaves
1 clove garlic
1 green onion, sliced
½ cup carrots, coarsely chopped
2 sprigs parsley
⅛ teaspoon sea salt
⅛ teaspoon freshly ground black pepper
½ cup boiling water

METHOD

Combine all ingredients in the blender adding the boiling water last.

Make sure the lid is secure and start at the lowest speed, gradually increasing to maximum speed.

Blend for at least two minutes until all ingredients are smooth and well blended.

Serve immediately.

SERVINGS: 2

It's Easy Being Green

Frothy and a lovely shade of green - yes, it's easy being green.

Ingredients

   ½ cup baby spinach, packed
   ½ cup kale, ribs removed, packed
   1 stalk celery, with leaves
   2 sprigs parsley
   1 large carrot, coarsely chopped
   1 green apple, coarsely chopped
   ½ cup water
   ½ cup ice cubes

Method

Place all ingredients in the blender.

Make sure the lid is secure and start at the lowest speed, gradually increasing to maximum speed.

Blend for at least one minute or until all ingredients are smooth and well blended.

Serve immediately.

Servings: 2

MINTY GREEN REFRESHER

The addition of mint to this drink makes all the difference. Very refreshing.

INGREDIENTS:

½ cup pineapple chunks
½ cup honeydew melon , chunks
2 spearmint leaves, or peppermint leaves
½ cup baby spinach, packed
½ cup kale, ribs removed, packed
½ cup water
½ cup ice cubes

METHOD:

Place all ingredients in the blender.

Make sure the lid is secure and start at the lowest speed, gradually increasing to maximum speed.

Blend for at least one minute or until all ingredients are smooth and well blended.

Serve immediately.

SERVINGS: 3

MULTI-BEAN SALAD

Why settle for a three-bean salad? This is our favorite, make-from-scratch, multi-bean salad! We like to make this the centerpiece of a large, salad supper.

We avoid using sugar whenever we can but to give this the traditional bean salad sweet/sour tang, we found it was necessary. We never use artificial sweeteners.

INGREDIENTS

   1½ cups kidney beans, cooked
   1½ cups chickpeas, cooked
   1 cup baby lima beans, cooked
   1 cup black beans, cooked
   1½ cups green beans, cooked, straight cut
   ½ medium red onion, diced
   2 stalks celery, diced
   ¼ medium green bell pepper, diced
   ¼ medium red bell pepper, diced
   2 garlic cloves, pressed
   ½ cup extra virgin olive oil
   ½ cup white vinegar
   ¼ cup balsamic vinegar
   ½ cup granulated sugar
   1½ teaspoons sea salt
   1 teaspoon black pepper, freshly ground

METHOD

All the beans in this recipe were cooked from dried beans with the exception, of course, of the green beans. They were cooked from fresh.

You can substitute canned beans in the recipe if it's easier for you. Just be sure to rinse the canned beans very well to eliminate any unwanted salt.

In a large glass bowl, combine all the beans, red onion, celery, and peppers.

Note: you don't want to use metal bowls when using vinegar. You could use plastic but glass works much better.

In a large measuring cup, combine the olive oil, vinegars, sugar, salt and pepper. Whisk well until ingredients are well combined and most of the sugar has dissolved.

Pour the oil and vinegar mixture over the bean mixture and stir well with a wooden spoon.

Cover the bean salad and refrigerate for at least 4 hours before serving. This allows all the flavors to blend and mature.

SERVINGS: 10

ORANGE, CARROT, APPLE JUICE

Simple and tasty with ingredients that are easy to find. It just takes a few minutes to make something that's really good for you. Go ahead, give it a try.

INGREDIENTS

1 medium orange, peeled
1 medium carrot, coarsely chopped
½ medium apple, coarsely chopped
1 cup pineapple chunks
½ cup water
½ cup ice cubes

METHOD

Place all ingredients in the blender.

Make sure the lid is secure and start at the lowest speed, gradually increasing to maximum speed.

Blend for at least one minute or until all ingredients are smooth and well blended.

Serve immediately.

SERVINGS: 2

Geoff & Vicky Wells

PEACHY GREEN SMOOTHIE

We all know that green tea is good for us. So, here's a recipe that also includes a lot of other good stuff. Almost a dessert this is so good.

INGREDIENTS

> 1 cup green tea, brewed and cooled
> ½ cup almond milk
> 2 peaches, pitted
> 1 frozen banana, cut in chunks
> 1½ tablespoons maple syrup, optional
> 1 cup ice cubes

METHOD

Place all the ingredients in your blender in the order given.

Make sure the lid is secure and start at the lowest speed, gradually increasing to maximum speed.

Blend for at least one minute or until all ingredients are smooth and well blended.

Serve immediately.

SERVINGS: 2

PEPPERED STRAWBERRIES

This is a wonderfully versatile recipe using strawberries - a favorite super food. You can serve this recipe, as-is, as either a dessert or an appetizer. You can also add these peppered strawberries to a salad as a colorful addition and an amazing taste experience. Or use them as a topping for your favorite dessert. The possibilities are endless - and delicious!

INGREDIENTS

> 1 pound fresh straweberries, rinsed and patted dry
> ¼ cup balsamic vinegar
> ¼ cup brown sugar
> 2 teaspoons black pepper, freshly ground

METHOD

Hull and quarter the strawberries and place them in a glass bowl.

In a glass measuring bowl, whisk together the vinegar and brown sugar until the sugar dissovles.

Pour the vinegar and sugar mixture over the strawberries and toss to coat evenly.

Grind the black pepper over the strawberries and toss again.

Serve or refrigerate immediately.

SERVINGS: 4

Geoff & Vicky Wells

RAW APPLE SAUCE

We like to use applesauce as a substitute for fats (oil, butter) in baked goods. Did you know you don't need to cook your apples to make your own, healthy applesauce? Try this recipe and you won't buy store bought applesauce again. We normally don't add the cinnamon or brown sugar.

INGREDIENTS

3 large apples
1½ teaspoons lemon juice, freshly squeezed
½ teaspoon cinnamon, optional
1 tablespoon brown sugar, optional

METHOD

Wash, core and quarter the apples. You can peel the apples if you like but we prefer not to. If you're using red apples, leaving the skins on gives the applesauce a rosy glow.

Add the apples, lemon juice, cinnamon (if using) and brown sugar (if using) to your blender.

Make sure the lid is secure and start at the lowest speed, gradually increasing to medium speed.

Be sure not to blend for too long, just long enough to get the proper applesauce consistency.

Transfer applesauce to an air tight container and refrigerate.

Use as desired.

SERVINGS: 4

RAW FRUIT SALAD

We love fresh fruit - love it! This is probably our best "How Many Super Foods Can You Stuff In A Recipe" recipe. Use this for breakfast or as a dessert. Enjoy!

INGREDIENTS

    1 cup strawberries, sliced
    ½ cup raspberries
    ½ cup blueberries
    1 kiwi, peeled and sliced
    1 nectarine, pitted and sliced
    1 sweet orange, peeled and chopped
    ½ cup pomegranate seeds
    1 small pear, seeded and chopped
    1 small apple, seeded
    ½ cup fresh pineapple chunks
    1 teaspoon black pepper, freshly ground
    ½ cup almonds, chopped
    ½ cup walnuts, chopped
    ½ cup coconut meat, freshly grated, optional

METHOD

Carefully rinse and dry all the fruit.

In a large bowl, combine all of the ingredients with the exception of the nuts and the coconut (if using).

Toss the ingredients gently to mix well. Cover and refrigerate for at least one hour before serving to allow the flavors to mix and a natural juice to form.

Just before serving, add the nuts and the coconut.

Note: you may just want to sprinkle the nuts and coconut on top of each serving.

SERVINGS: 12

RAW VEGGIES AND DIP

This is a very simple recipe but one that, we've found, most people don't tend to do. This is a great idea for your evening meal. Who says the vegetables have to be cooked just because it's suppertime?

INGREDIENTS

4 stalks celery
2 medium carrots
½ head cauliflower
1 head broccoli
4 spring onions
½ medium cucumber
½ medium red bell pepper
½ cup sugar snap peas
½ cup fresh green beans
1 cup hummus, for dip

METHOD

Clean all of the vegetables and cut into bite-size pieces.

We like to vary how we cut them up and do things like cut the carrots into matchsticks, the cauliflower and broccoli into flowerets, the cucumber into spears - you get the idea.

Provide each person with their own small dish of hummus to use as a dip.

That's it - easy and healthy!

SERVINGS: 4

RICE MILK

Yes, it is possible - and easy - to make your our rice milk with this simple recipe. Although we've shown the brown sugar and vanilla as optional, we prefer it made that way.

INGREDIENTS

½ cup brown rice, cooked
2 cups filtered water
1½ teaspoons brown sugar, optional
½ teaspoon vanilla, optional

METHOD

Place all ingredients in the blender.

Make sure the lid is secure and begin blending at lowest speed increasing gradually to maximum speed.

Blend for at least two minutes or until smooth.

Store in the refrigerator and be sure to shake well before using.

SERVINGS: 4

Spicy Tomato Juice

Want a little "kick" in your tomato juice? This recipe certainly provides that.

Ingredients

    2 cups tomatoes, coarsely chopped
    ¼ medium green bell pepper
    1 green onion, sliced
    1 clove garlic
    ½ jalapeno pepper, seeded and chopped
    1 dash sea salt, optional
    1 dash freshly ground black pepper, optional

Method

Place all ingredients in the blender.

Make sure the lid is secure and start at the lowest speed, gradually increasing to maximum speed.

Blend for at least one minute or until all ingredients are smooth and well blended.

Serve immediately or chill for later use.

Servings: 3

TASTY GREEN SALAD

A quick and easy salad. If you grow your own greens, so much the better. If not, try to find the freshest ones available and use them right away.

INGREDIENTS

> 1 medium red apple, seeded and chopped
> 2 tablespoons extra virgin olive oil
> ¼ teaspoon fresh lemon peel, grated
> 1 tablespoon fresh lemon juice
> 2 teaspoons apple cider vinegar
> 2 teaspoons red onion, minced
> 1 teaspoon maple syrup
> 8 cups mixed greens, (romaine, arugula, spinach, kale, etc.)
> freshly ground black pepper, to taste

METHOD

After chopping the apple, toss it in a little lemon juice to prevent browning.

Wash the greens, rinse well and spin or pat dry. Place them in a large salad bowl and set aside.

In a large measuring cup, whisk together the olive oil, lemon peel, lemon juice, vinegar, red onion and maple syrup. Then mix the apples into this dressing.

Gently pour the dressing over the mixed greens and toss to coat.

Grind the black pepper on the top, to taste, and serve immediately.

SERVINGS: 4

TOMATO, CUCUMBER AND CILANTRO SALAD

Tasty, filling and super-low in calories.

INGREDIENTS

   4 medium ripe tomatoes, cut in wedges
   1 large English cucumber, sliced
   ½ medium red onion, chopped
   ½ medium green bell pepper, chopped
   2 cloves garlic, minced
   ¼ cup fresh cilantro, chopped
   2 tablespoons balsamic vinegar
   sea salt, to taste
   black pepper, freshly ground, to taste

METHOD

In a large bowl, combine all the ingredients and gently toss to coat.

Cover and refrigerate for at least 1/2 hour to allow the flavors to blend.

Serve on a bed of lettuce. Add more salt and pepper, if desired.

SERVINGS: 4

Very Berry Smoothie

Can you have too many berries? We sure don't think so. These super foods are tasty, sweet and really, really good for you.

Try it without the maple syrup first. We sure find it sweet enough that way.

Ingredients

 1½ cups almond milk
 ½ cup blueberries, fresh or frozen
 ½ cup strawberries, fresh or frozen
 ½ cup raspberries, fresh or frozen
 ½ cup blackberries, fresh or frozen
 1 medium banana, fresh or frozen
 1 tablespoon ground flax seed
 2 tablespoons maple syrup, optional
 1 cup ice cubes

Method

Place all the ingredients in your blender in the order given.

Make sure the lid is secure and start at the lowest speed, gradually increasing to maximum speed.

Blend for at least one minute or until all ingredients are smooth and well blended.

Serve immediately.

Servings: 4

VICKY'S FAVORITE BREAKFAST SMOOTHIE

If you're using just a regular blender (we use a VitaMix) you'll need to cut things up fairly small. For a commercial grade blender, large-size chunks are fine.

INGREDIENTS

    1 cup almond milk
    1½ cups water
    ½ large cucumber, peeled
    2 large carrots, peeled
    1 medium apple, cored and sliced
    1 small banana, frozen
    1 medium pear, cored and sliced
    ½ inch ginger, piece, peeled
    3 cups garden greens, packed - kale, spinach, lettuce, etc.
    2 tablespoons maple syrup, optional

METHOD

Place all of the ingredients in the blender in the order they are listed.

Note: I put half of the greens in until they get blended down somewhat and then added the rest.

Make sure that lid is secure and begin blending at lowest speed increasing gradually to maximum speed.

Blend for at least one minute or until everything is well blended and smooth.

Serve immediately.

SERVINGS: 3

VICKY'S GRANOLA

Okay, this recipe isn't raw, but it's very healthy. Sometimes switching to plant based can make you feel a little confused and wishing for something familiar. This is very tasty and so much better than any packaged cereal. Be sure to have it with almond or coconut milk.

INGREDIENTS

> 4 cups rolled oats, old fashioned, not quick or minute
> ½ cup ground flax seed
> ½ cup oat bran
> ½ cup wheat germ
> ½ cup sunflower seeds
> ½ cup almonds, chopped
> ½ cup walnuts, chopped
> ½ teaspoon sea salt
> ½ cup brown sugar
> ½ cup maple syrup
> ⅓ cup coconut oil
> 2 teaspoons ground cinnamon
> 1½ teaspoons vanilla extract
> 1 cup raisins and/or sweetened dried cranberries

METHOD

Pre-heat the oven to 325° F and lightly grease a large baking sheet.

Combine the oats, flax seed, oat bran, sunflower seeds, almonds and walnuts in a large bowl.

In a small saucepan, mix together the salt, brown sugar, maple syrup, coconut oil, cinnamon and vanilla. Over medium heat, bring the mixture to a boil and remove from heat.

Pour the liquid mixture over the oat mixture and stir well to coat everything evenly. Then spread the mixture evenly on the greased baking sheet.

Bake at 325° F for 20 minutes, Remove from the oven and allow to cool.

Add the raisins and/or cranberries and stir.

Note: after baking mixture can get quite hard, you may have to break it up.

Store completed granola in an airtight container.

SERVINGS: 12

Zesty Cucumber Salad

A refreshing cucumber salad with a bit of a kick. Be sure NOT to peel the cucumbers. You want all the nutrients that are in the skin.

For a more interesting look, score the length of each cucumber with a fork before slicing.

Ingredients

2 large English cucumbers, sliced
2 teaspoons sea salt
¼ cup white vinegar
¼ cup balsamic vinegar
¼ cup sugar
2 tablespoons extra virgin olive oil
2 cloves garlic, minced
1 tablespoon fresh ginger, grated
4 slices jalapeno pepper, minced

Method

Place the sliced cucumbers in a colander and sprinkle them with the sea salt.

Place the colander in a glass bowl (to catch any liquid) and allow to drain in the refrigerator for one hour.

In a separate glass bowl, whisk together the vinegars and sugar until the sugar has dissolved. The add the olive oil, garlic, ginger and jalapeño. Stir well.

Remove the cucumber slices from the refrigerator and rinse off the salt with cold water. Place the slices in a large bowl and pour the oil and vinegar mixture over them. Toss to coat.

Serve immediately.

Servings: 6

ALMOST WALDORF SALAD (NO MAYO)

Waldorf salad is, of course, a classic. In this take we've eliminated the mayonnaise and replaced it with hummus. If you need to thin the hummus a bit, just add a little lemon juice and olive oil to achieve the desired consistency.

INGREDIENTS

1 medium red apple, cored and chopped
1 teaspoon lemon juice, freshly squeezed
½ cup walnuts, chopped
½ cup celery, sliced
½ cup seedless grapes, halved
¼ cup hummus
sea salt, to taste
black pepper, to taste
2-3 cups mixed baby greens

METHOD

Toss the chopped apple in the lemon juice to prevent browning.

In a large bowl, combine all the chopped apple, walnuts, celery and grapes. Mix in the hummus and make sure everything is well coated.

Add salt and pepper to taste and serve over a bed of mixed greens.

SERVINGS: 2

Nut Butter

This is likely to be one of the easiest, shortest recipes you're likely to see. One ingredient! One direction!

Our favorite nuts to use are almonds, peanuts or cashews. You can also make a combination if you like.

You can use either a blender or a food processor. We used a Vitamix. However, be aware that not all blenders or food processors can handle this process.

Ingredients

    3 cups nuts of your choice, roasted or raw

Method

Place the nuts in your blender or food processor and process until you achieve the right consistency.

Yep, that's it!

Servings: 6

SPICY LETTUCE WRAPS

This is lovely for a snack or as the focal point of a light lunch. If you're allergic to peanuts you can substitute just about any other nut. Be sure to let the filling marinate so that the flavors and blend and mature.

INGREDIENTS:

    2 medium carrots, grated
    1 medium zucchini, grated
    1 rib celery, minced
    ¼ cup peanuts, chopped
    2 teaspoons fresh ginger, grated
    ½ teaspoon tabasco sauce
    2 teaspoons sesame oil
    1 tablespoon soy sauce
    2 teaspoons lime juice
    lettuce leaves, washed, rinsed and dried

METHOD:

In a glass bowl, combine all of the ingredients, with the exception of the lettuce leaves, and mix well. Cover and refrigerate for at least one hour - overnight is better.

Drain any excess liquid from the vegetable mixture. Place just enough of the vegetable mixture in each lettuce leaf so that you can fold the leaf into a packet. The number of wraps you get will depend the size of the lettuce leaves and how much filling you use in each one.

If necessary, secure each lettuce wrap with a toothpick and serve immediately.

Note: you can use any type of lettuce leaf but we find that iceberg lettuce is the easiest to work with in this recipe.

SERVINGS: 2

ABOUT THE AUTHORS

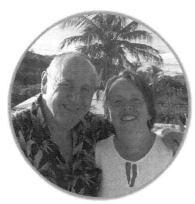

Geoff Wells and his wife, Vicky, were not the healthiest people when they first got married. They lived hectic lifestyles and opted, on many nights, to settle for something that was quick and easy, rather than something healthy and nutritious. When health issues, and weight gain, started to manifest, they decided that a more healthy solution had to found.

They started to do their research and came upon the idea of juicing. It provided a healthy alternative to their current food choices and they found that juicing took very little time. So their weight loss adventure began but they also wanted to be sure that they were keeping everything in balance. After all, it wasn't just about weight loss but healthy eating, too. After additional research they found out about raw foods and Superfoods.

After seeing the positive results from modifying their diet they made the decision to share what they had learned with all who were interested. Geoff and Vicky believe they have found the key to living a healthy lifestyle and are proud to share what they know thus far. It is simple to follow and they have provided a large number of recipes to make switching to this type of lifestyle even easier.

PLEASE REVIEW

I hope you have enjoyed this book and will post a favorable review. Independent authors rely on feedback from readers like you to spread the word about books you enjoy. You can leave your comments and contact the author directly by visiting the Geezer Guides web site.

Geezer Guides (the publisher of this book) frequently promotes new titles by offering free copies on special one day only sales. As one of my readers I would like you to get all my new books without charge. Just visit http://ebooks.geezerguides.com and get on their mailing list by filling out the simple form there.

OTHER BOOKS FROM GEEZER GUIDES

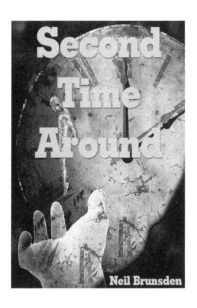

http://ebooks.geezerguides.com/book/second-
time-around/

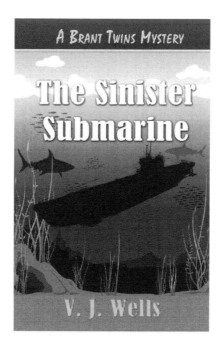

http://ebooks.geezerguides.com/book/the-sinister-submarine/

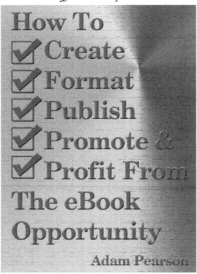

http://ebooks.geezerguides.com/book/how-to-create-format-publish-promote-profit-from-the-ebook-opportunity/

Made in the USA
San Bernardino, CA
14 October 2013